REPAIR

For Toddlers

A Children's Program for Recovery from Incest and Childhood Sexual Abuse

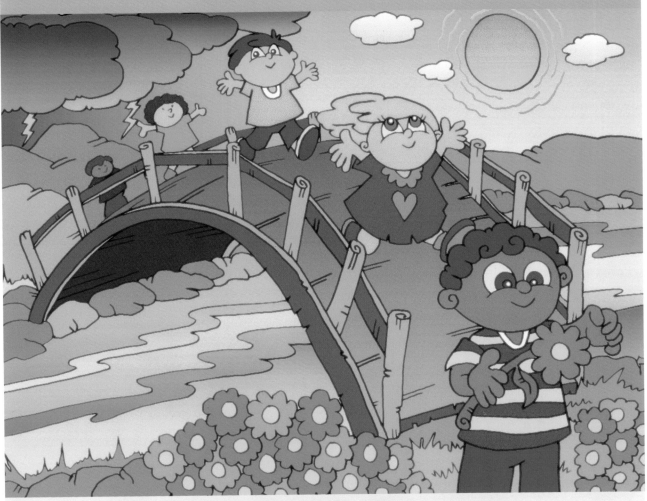

Marjorie McKinnon

Illustrated by Tom W. McKinnon

Repair For Toddlers: A Children's Program for Recovery from Incest and Childhood Sexual Abuse.
From the *Growing with Love* Series.
Copyright © 2011 by Marjorie McKinnon and Tom W. McKinnon. All Rights Reserved.
First Edition: January 2011

Learn more about the McKinnons at www.TheLampLighters.org

Library of Congress Cataloging-in-Publication Data

McKinnon, Margie, 1942-
  Repair for toddlers : a children's program for recovery from incest & childhood sexual abuse / By Marjorie McKinnon ; illustrated by Tom W. McKinnon. -- 1st ed.
       p. cm.
  Includes bibliographical references and index.
  ISBN-13: 978-1-61599-089-4 (trade paper : alk. paper)
  ISBN-10: 1-61599-089-5 (trade paper : alk. paper)
  1. Sexually abused children--Rehabilitation. 2. Incest victims--Rehabilitation. 3. Toddlers--Mental health. I. Title.
  RJ507.S49M383 2011
  618.92'85836--dc22
                                    2010047483

Special Thanks to: Melanie Doty for helping me put this together

Distributed by:
Baker & Taylor, Ingram Book Group, New Leaf Distributing

Published by:
Loving Healing Press
5145 Pontiac Trail
Ann Arbor, MI 48105
USA

www.LovingHealing.com or
info@LovingHealing.com
Phone 888 761 6268
Fax +1 734 663 6861

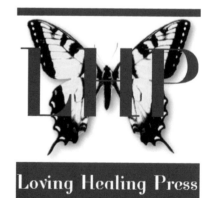

Loving Healing Press

To my beloved grandchildren ......

And grandchildren everywhere

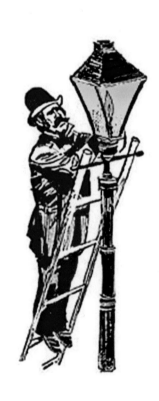

Instructions for the Caregiver

This book is designed to help children from ages two to six who have been sexually abused. While some people have a problem believing that children of those ages could be sexually abused, it happens more frequently than you'd like to hear. Just ask your local Child Protective Services for information on how often they confront it. We intend to convert the original REPAIR program so that this book can be used to help toddlers, that is from ages two to six, who have been violated.

Start by reading this book to yourself so that you can be familiar with the technique. Since your child won't be able to read, you will be reading it to them as you go along. You will point out the different illustrations and talk about them and what they mean. Some children, depending on their age, will be able to grasp it sooner than others.

Keep in mind that all children who have been sexually abused (or other abused in other ways) feel very bad about themselves. Since they can't read this book and it will be difficult for them even to talk about what happened to them, you must put yourself in their position through Imagination, Compassion, and Solutions. In *Imagination* you must try to imagine what might have happened sexually to that child. Perhaps you remember an incident that happened to you. Picture yourself as a two or three year old. Picture your body being violated in a way that is painful, shameful and unfortunately might also be enjoyable but is nevertheless violated. The only thing a child knows when they are sexually abused is that they must not talk about it. Even if no one said, "Don't tell," there is something about what happened to them that is so shameful that they pretend it never happened. But it's all there, in that closet in their mind. Next you must treat them with *Compassion.* Here you will utilize skills that will show that you care, that you can emphasize, that you feel sorrow at what happened. In *Solution* you will utilize different techniques and exercises that will take them from a place of dark despair to joy. You will use the "Bridge of Recovery" to explain to them what will happen. Set aside a certain amount of time as often as you can to play with your child the game called REPAIR. Tell them it will help them feel wonderful about themselves and will chase away the demons that caused them to feel bad.

At that age they are capable of talking, of expressing their own wants and ideas. They are also capable of expressing their own pains. Some will be more verbal than others.

I encourage you to call 425.226.5062. It's the phone number for the King County Sexual Assault Resource Center in Renton, WA. Request them to mail you a copy of the brochure titled "He Told Me Not To Tell". It's a parent's guide to talking to children about sexual assault and it's an awesome resource. It is totally free and they will mail you as many copies as you need. The brochure contains ideas that will give you additional help.

A word to the Caregiver…. Loneliness may come to you as you help your child but in using this book, you too will be REPAIRED. This was not your fault either. Thank you for taking the courage to work with your child.

Like the book *REPAIR For Kids: A Children's Program for Recovery from Incest and Childhood Sexual Abuse*, *REPAIR For Toddlers* is also based on the word REPAIR which is an acronym for the stages of the program. They are:

R – Recognition: where the child will come to realize that someone bad did something bad to them and that it's okay to talk about it

E – Entry: where you explain to the child that they will be playing the REPAIR game on a regular basis and that it will ultimately take the bad times out of their head and guide them to a place of joy.

P – Process: as the child crosses from one side of the Bridge of Recovery to the other side they will be using tools to help them get there. These tools are all in this part of the program.

A – Awareness: where once the tools have been implemented and maintained on a regular basis the child comes to realize that it was not their fault.

I – Insight: where the child sees the big picture wherein they discover they were only a pawn on a chess board.

R – Rhythm where the child learns to return to that joyful promise made at their birth, the promise that allows them to be who they really are, the promise that was ripped away from them when they were abused.

Let's start this program with the word *REPAIR* and an explanation to the child regarding what it means.

HELLO LITTLE ONE
We are going to play a game!

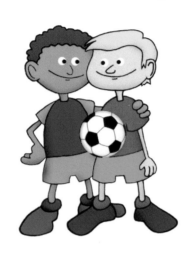

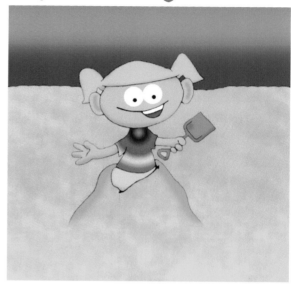

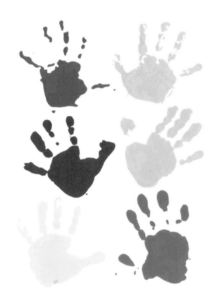

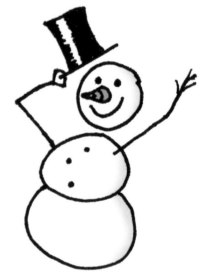

No, it's not like any of these.
We are going to use this book

A Children's Program for Recovery

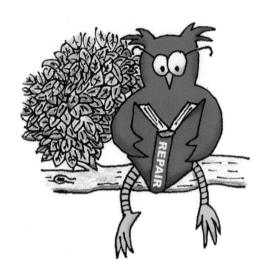

to play the game called

REPAIR

It means to fix something that's broken, like they're doing in these pictures.

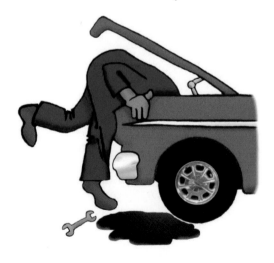

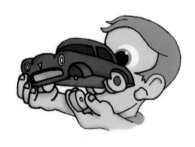

When we were born we were given a promise, a promise that we would have the tools we need to live a joyful life.

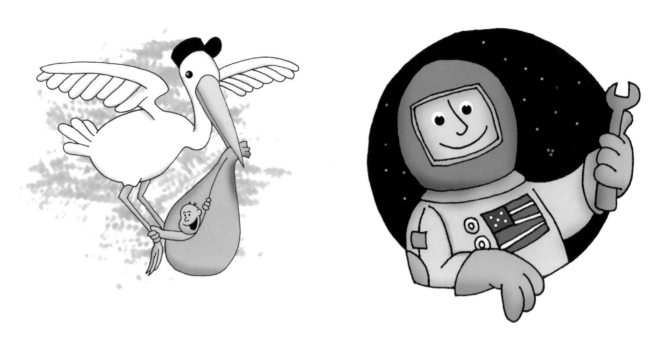

Then something happened to <u>us</u>

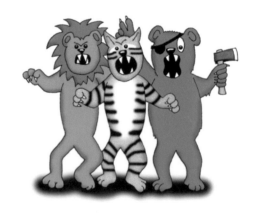

And we became fearful
Like the lion and tiger and bear did in
"The Wizard of Oz"

A Children's Program for Recovery

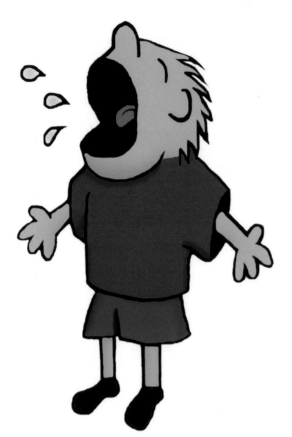

We became a
wounded child.

But we can be REPAIRED.
LET'S PLAY OUR GAME!!
The first LETTER in the game,

REPAIR

IS R for

RECOGNITION

(I know, I know it's a BIG word)

Let's start with some questions.
Are you sad a lot of the time? I know you can't answer me but you can tell whoever is helping you with this program whether you are sad or not.

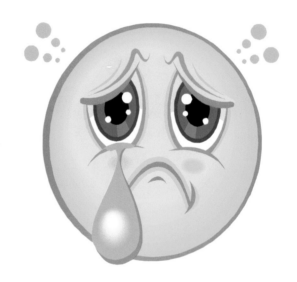

Do you feel like someone made you do something lately that made you feel "yucky?

Or even asked you to do something that made you feel "funny", not funny in a good way, but funny in a bad way?

Do you feel like the "happy" you has changed to the "sad" you?

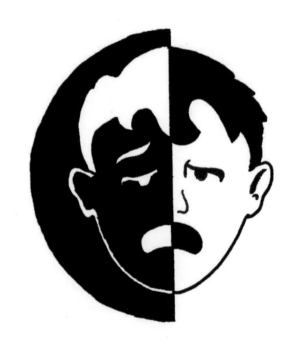

Do you cry a lot?

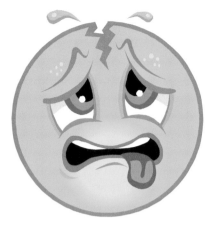

But don't know why?

If your answer to any of these questions is yes, then you should tell the person who's helping you to REPAIR exactly what happened. No matter what the person—who did the yucky things to you—said, even if they told you not to tell, they were wrong. It is ok to tell whoever is helping you with this game exactly what happened.

Now we are going to do something that will be fun. It will help us feel better.

We are going to cross a bridge.

Let's make believe this is the bridge we are going to cross.
It is the MAGICAL BRIDGE OF RECOVERY!!!

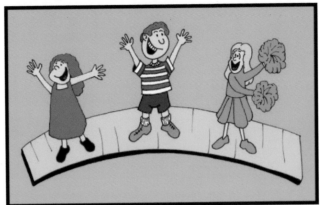

On this side of the bridge a lot of confusing things have happened, things that didn't feel good, that made you wonder if you were okay. A part of you didn't want to talk about it. You became

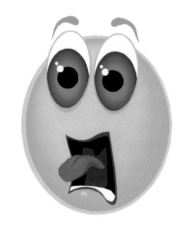
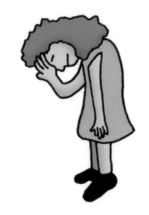
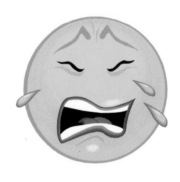

Fearful   *sad and felt shame,*   *cried a lot*

and *couldn't trust anyone anymore.*

BUT - On the other side of the bridge are all kinds of good things.

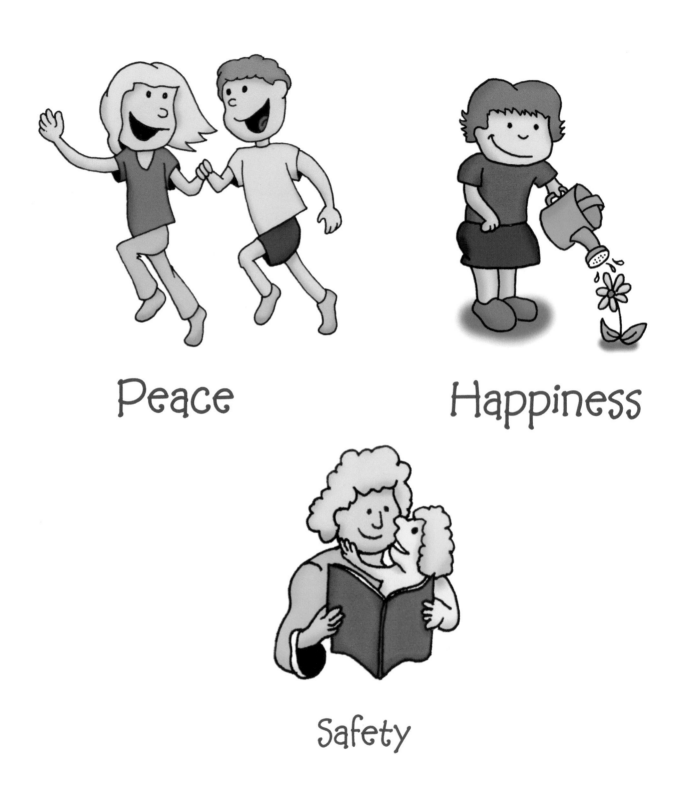

Peace

Happiness

Safety

A Children's Program for Recovery

We have one more part to the big word, Recognition
We're going to learn what belongs to us and what doesn't.

Let's start by talking about body parts.

This is your ear

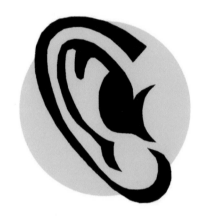

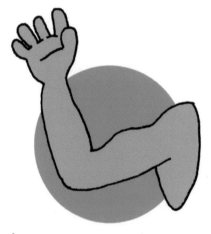

This is your arm

Let's do some more...

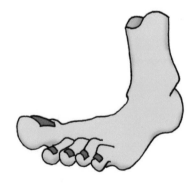

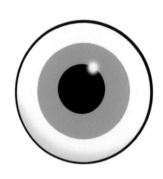

Your foot...   Your eye...

But we also have some very private parts to our body.

The part between our legs, where we go little potty with, is called our penis (if you are a boy) and vagina (if you are a girl).

Your mouth is another private part.

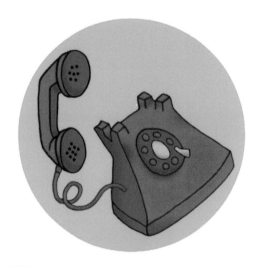

You don't have to put anything in your mouth that makes you uncomfortable. If anyone tries to put something in your mouth that you don't want there you can call 911 and tell them you need help.

The place where all of the private body parts are located is either in the genital (little potty) or the anal (big potty) area.

One more is in the breast area on your chest where the two brown circles are. They are called nipples.

It is okay if we call our body parts what they are.

These body parts belong to us and no one can touch them. If someone ever tries to trick you, confuse you or hurt you again, promise yourself you will follow this rule: You will TELL, TELL, TELL. There are healthy adults who can help you and protect you. If you don't know of any,

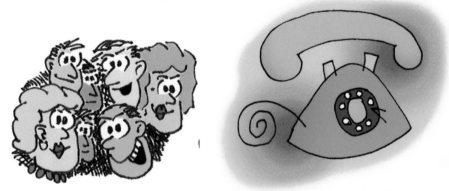

remember to pick up the phone and dial 911. Your caregiver will show you how to do this. You can learn to trust again, and trust your feelings. Here's another example of what belongs to us. This is YOUR toy.

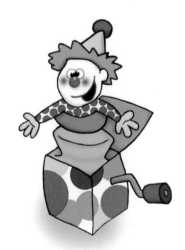

This is <u>Daddy's</u> wallet.

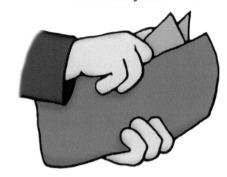

We can play with <u>our</u> toy, but we mustn't take anything out of <u>Daddy's</u> wallet.

This also means no one can touch us in our private places because they are ours. If anyone tries to touch us in our private places we feel it must be our fault. But no one has the right to touch any part of our body that we don't want them to. It is not OUR fault. It is THEIR fault.

> If that happens, we must tell someone whom we feel safe with right away. Remember 911.

Sometimes the person who touched our private parts is someone in our family. But they still do not have any right to touch us there.

We are going to learn in this book how to REPAIR ourselves if this has happened to us, sort of like getting a band-aid put on when we have an owie or like going to the doctor when we're sick.

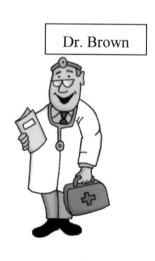

Dr. Brown

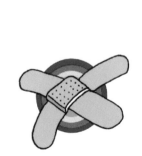

A Children's Program for Recovery

Now we are going to do the next thing in the game, the game of REPAIR in which we will cross a bridge and get to the good things on the other side.

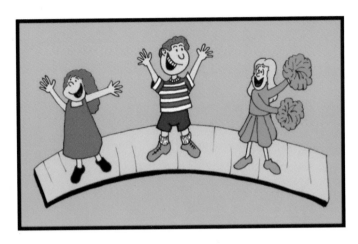

ENTRY is the next part of the game.

See... it's the E in

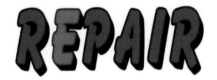

It means "to make a beginning".

It's sort of like opening a door.

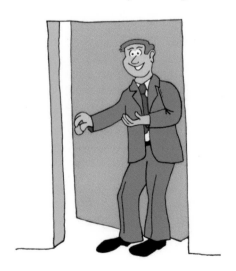

We are going to promise ourselves to do this REPAIR game, both of us together as often as we can. That's sort of what entry means.

> Other children that have had this happen are going across the bridge too. You are not alone.

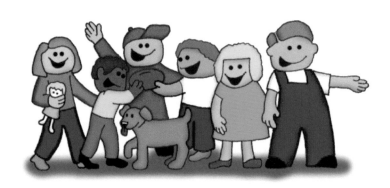

The next letter in **REPAIR** is $\underline{P}$

It means PROCESS

This is the fun part of the game.

First, let's try the game called *What am I feeling?*

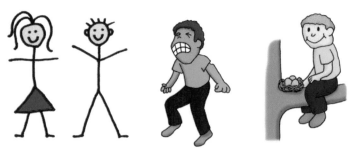

You can be happy, angry, excited,

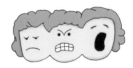

sad angry, very unhappy.

A Children's Program for Recovery

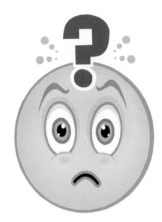

You can be confused.

But it's important to Know what you are feeling. Every time you work on REPAIR be sure to say what you are feeling. Next, we are going to do the Magic Mirror game.

This one is FUN!

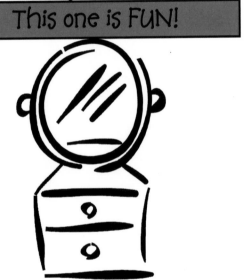

Here is a mirror. We are going to look into the mirror and say as many good things about ourselves as we can. Let's see how many we can think of. Here's a few to get you started.

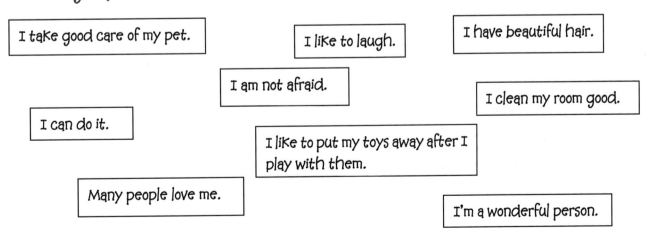

I take good care of my pet.

I like to laugh.

I have beautiful hair.

I am not afraid.

I clean my room good.

I can do it.

I like to put my toys away after I play with them.

Many people love me.

I'm a wonderful person.

Now we can say: "Mirror, Mirror on the wall,
Who's the fairest of them all?"

WE ARE! WE ARE!

We are going to do this every day!

There is an inner you that knows the truth of what happened. Sometimes, when we think about it, we get really scared. That inner child is waiting with a sad face for us to set her free, to tell her story to someone she feels safe with.

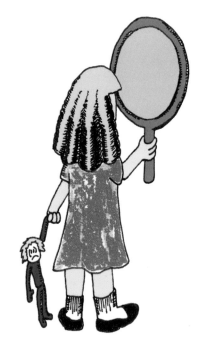

It might help if we had a special toy or a doll that we could hold while we were looking into the magic mirror.

Here's some!!!

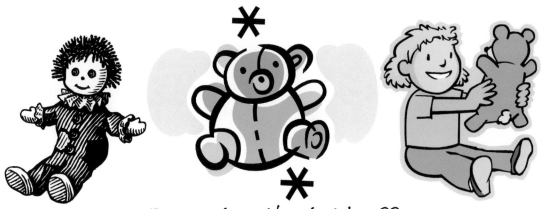

Remember the bridge??

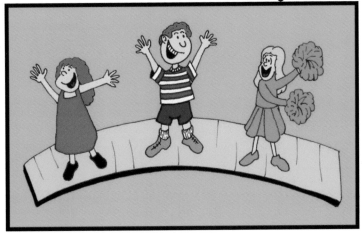

We're halfway across it. Now let's talk about bad things people say to us, like:

| You're so stupid. | Let's change that to: | I'm so smart! |
| Stop that crying! | Let's change that to: | I am sad!! |

Can you think of some more bad things you hear that you can change to good things?

We all have "stinker" qualities. We may not be perfect but we are really, really good. Sometimes when we are sad we want to fight with our little brother. Some days we get out of bed on the wrong side.....like this little boy did.

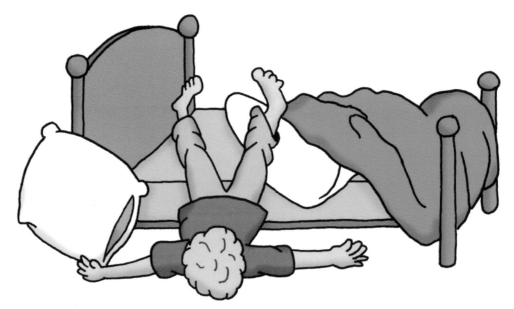

   This may be because someone touched our bodies in a way that made us feel sad and yucky. But these stinker qualities don't belong to us. They belong to the person that touched our bodies when they weren't supposed to. So whenever we feel a stinker quality coming on we should say what they are, like "I feel cranky today." We can choose our feelings if we don't like the ones we have.

   We can throw away any bad words anyone said to us, like this lady did below. We don't agree!

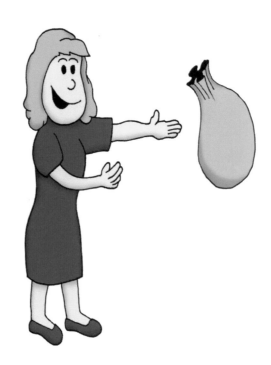

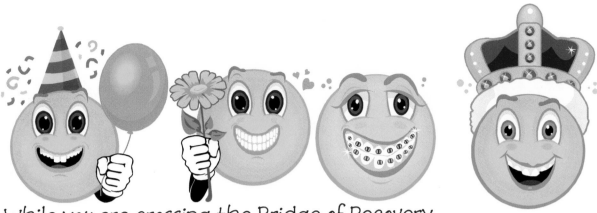

While you are crossing the Bridge of Recovery
You might need some help. Say HALT to yourself.
That means Take care of yourself when you are feeling:

Hungry
Angry
Lonely
Tired

And you will soon feel better!!!

For example: Hungry – eat peanut butter and jelly sandwich

Angry – I will punch my pillow ten times.

Lonely – I will hug my pet or have a sleepover with a friend.

Tired – I will take a nap.

Think of four of each

The Attitude of Gratitude

Say several things that you are grateful for. No matter how small. For example: "I have a great bedroom," "My grandma and I are real close, I am so grateful for her," "I love my hair; it's long and curly," and so on.

Courage Songs

This part is going to be fun. Think of any songs you know that you like to sing, that make you feel better when you sing them. How about: "It's A Small World After All" for starters?

Pamper yourself!

Do something special for yourself that is fun: Play an extra fun game, eat popcorn while you watch a Disney movie, look at the pictures in a happy book, ride your bike, have a bubble bath. Think of some yourself. It's like giving a gift to yourself.

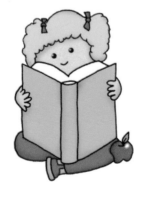 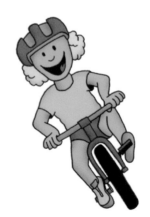 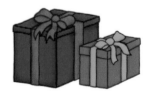

Now
We learn how to set boundaries.

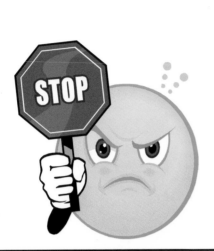 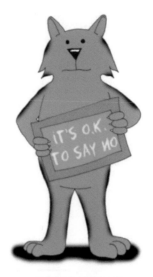

It's like putting up a stop sign or a fence telling people they can't touch us. Practice saying "no". Say it over and over. Have the person who is helping you with this game play-act on how to say "no". You are setting new boundaries.

Next comes the **A** part of REPAIR.

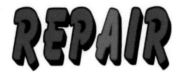

It's a big word, **AWARENESS**, but you can call it the "magic word". It is "magic" because it means "smart" you. Remember when you learned how to throw a ball, eat with a spoon, color with crayons, go potty on your own.

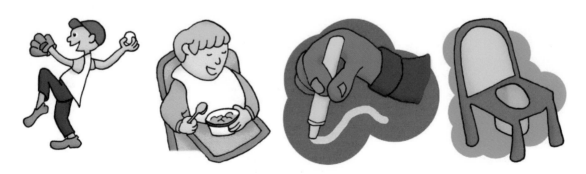

We felt so smart! And we were! How about if we smelled chocolate baking in the kitchen? We guessed that mom was baking a cake. That's because we're using the magical word that means "smart". And we are learning something even better. We are opening doors and learning the word TRUTH. When a person wants us to touch their private body parts or wants to touch ours we will TELL TELL TELL the

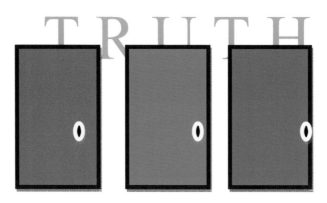

We are becoming stronger. We know now that if someone hurts us, it isn't our fault. It is their fault. If <u>anyone</u> touches us in a place we don't want to be touched we can scream our heads off or dial 911 for the police who'll help us. People are waiting to help us.

We now know we have the right to say "no". This magical word, Awareness, which means <u>SMART YOU</u>, is a wonderful thing.

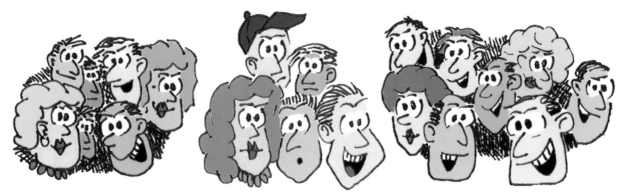

The Good Guys!!

Now let's go to the letter I in

REPAIR

It means **INSIGHT,** but you can call it "looking in". It is another magical word.

So here you are, crossing that bridge and you realize you're more than halfway across. Do something fun to celebrate.

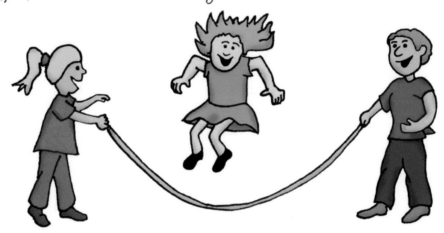

Here we are going to play two different games. One is called "Real Love Qualities". Here we tell whoever is working this game with us what kind of "real love" qualities we'd like to receive from our parents/caregivers. Like maybe, "I want to bake cookies with you", or "Can I to go to the park more often?" or, "Can you give me a hug?" Say at least one a day. We might need a little push to help us with this. But it's important. We need what's called "NURTURING". It's a big word that means to take care of us, to give us love, and make us feel loved.

The next game is to talk about your wonderful qualities. See how many you can say, like: "I have pretty eyes", "I like my long blonde hair", "I like animals", and so on. Try to say some every time you work this part of the game.

Now for the last letter of this game, which is R. It stands for RHYTHM.

REPAIR

Rhythm is a very special word. Do you know how to dance? Dance for a few minutes, or if you like to play ball do that.

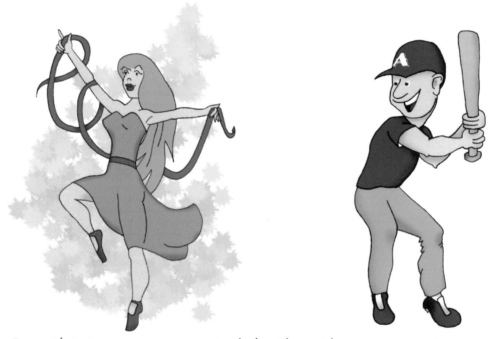

See, this is your own magical rhythm, the way you dance or play ball.

But, before someone did things to you that made you feel yucky, you had that rhythm that was just YOU! It went away when the bad person did something they were not supposed to do; something that was wrong and bad and that we had to tell someone we feel safe with.

When someone hurt that private part of us that we spoke of earlier or if they made us feel bad by making us take our clothes off when we didn't want to, we lost that special dance we had, the one that was just like us and no one else. If we liked climbing trees, now we felt sad every time we passed a tree.

But guess what!
We have been moving across the bridge...

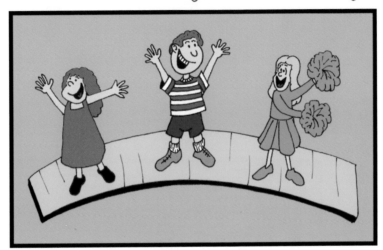

Every day we have been returning to our own RHYTHM, our own dance, the one that was ripped away from us when someone did something bad to us.

Now we are going to play a very important game. It's called,

"Who Am I?"

Say out loud all the things you are. Are you playful? Do you giggle? Do you like playing in the sand at the beach, or do you like going to the woods instead? How about animals? Do you like puppies or kittens or maybe both? Leave nothing out. Every time you play the REPAIR game and you come to this part, say everything you can think of.

Now for the last most wonderful game of all, "MY WISH LIST".

This is like Christmas when Santa Claus comes. Say all the things you'd like to be, to have, or to do. Do you want long hair? Do you want to be a doctor when you grow up? Do you want Grandpa to visit? Or do you want a dog or a cat? If you picture something you want, you just might get it... if you're patient!!!

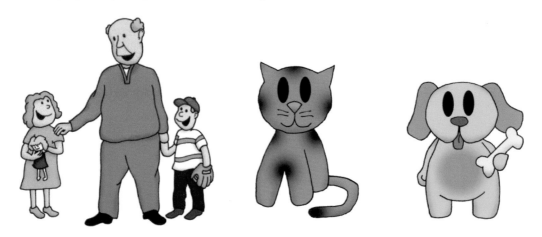

Now you have played the REPAIR game perfectly. You have crossed the bridge. Hooray!

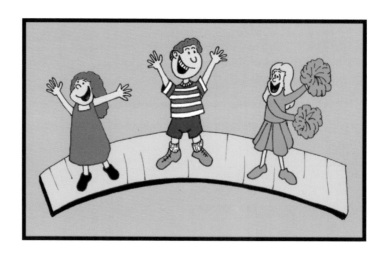

That child inside of you has taken all the bad things that happened to you and thrown them in the trash can.

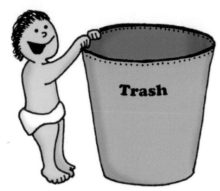

You have gone from being a ghost of your former self,

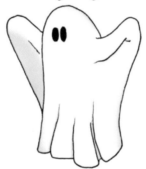

To being the real you, happy and not afraid.

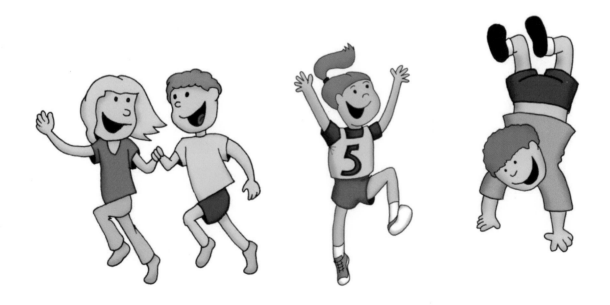

You have learned that no one can tell you, "NOT TO TELL"; no one can do yucky things to your body again. You can dial 911 if they even try.

You are now strong and powerful and you have learned the game

REPAIR

Jump for joy!!

Wag your tail!!

Take a bow!

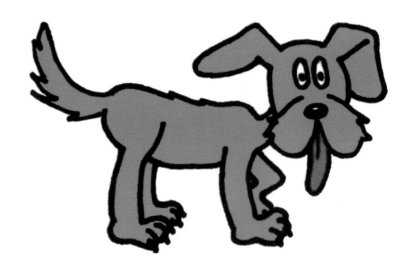

HOORAY FOR YOU!

You are absolutely wonderful.

You now have a chance to go from being afraid and ashamed to being a joyful, stable child. You now know that you can TELL no matter who tells you not to.....

TELL TELL TELL

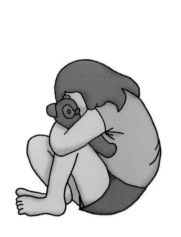
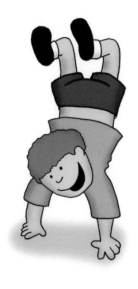
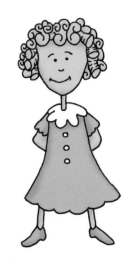

You have a chance to live happily ever after, with the help of the REPAIR game and the ones who nurture you, respect you and take good care of you.

Stay smart, stay safe. Play safe,

Be silly and have FUN

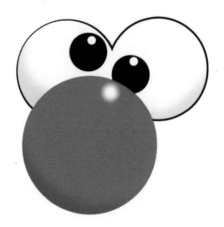

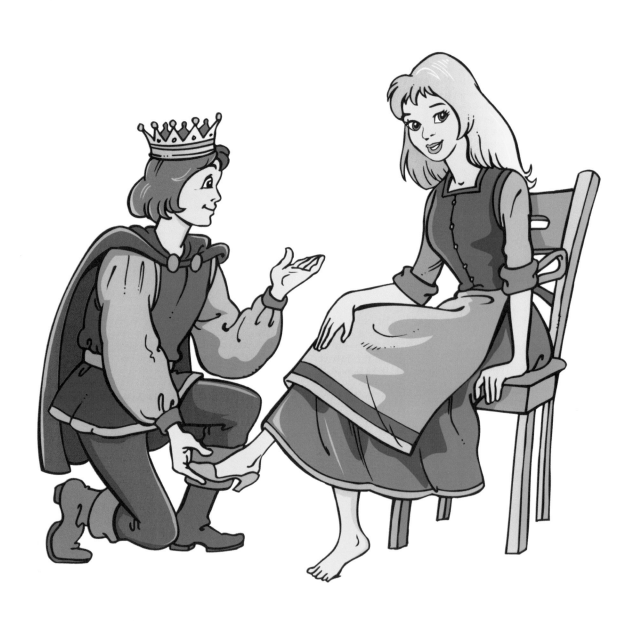

The Serenity Prayer
(children's version)

(We have included the children's version of The Serenity Prayer. Please help your child to memorize it and say it often, especially when they are feeling sad.)

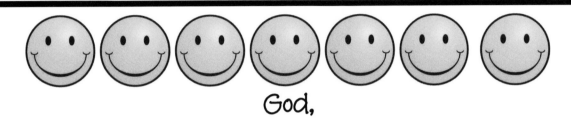

God,

Please make me calm,

So I can accept things,

I cannot change,

Make me brave,

So I can change things I can,

And make me smart enough,

To know the difference.

Amen

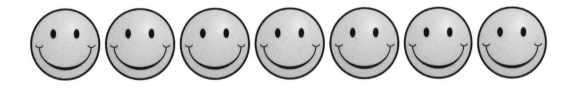

Suggested Reading

- *Bullies Are A Pain in the Brain,* by Trevor Romain and Elizabeth Verdick (age 9-12)

- *Cool Cats, Calm Kids: Relaxation and Stress Management for Young People*, by Mary L. Williams, illustrated by Dianne O'Quinn Burke (age 7–12)

- *Don't Rant and Rave on Wednesdays: The Children's Anger-Control Book*, by Adolph Moser, illustrated by David Melton (age 9-12)

- *Don't Feed the Monsters on Tuesdays: The Children's Self-Esteem Book*, by Adolph Moser (age 9-12)

- *Don't Pop Your Cork on Mondays: The Children's Anti-Stress Book*, by Adolph Moser, illustrated by Dave Pilkey (age 9-12)

- *Let's Talk About – Feeling Angry,* by Joy Wilt Berry, illustrated by Maggie Smith (age 4-8)

- *Let's Talk About – Feeling Sad,* by Joy Wilt Berry (age 4-8)

- *Let's Talk About – Needing Attention,* by Joy Wilt Berry (age 4-8)

- *Let's Talk About – Saying No,* by Joy Wilt Berry (age 4-8)

- *Psychology for Kids: 40 Fun Tests That Help You Learn About Yourself,* by Jonni Kinder and Julie S. Buck (age 9-12)

- *Stick Up For Yourself: Every Kid's Guide to Personal Power and Positive Self-Esteem,* by Gershen Kaufman and Lev Raphael (age 9-12)

- *What Do You Think: A Kid's Guide to Dealing with Daily Dilemmas,* by Linda Schwartz and Beverly Armstrong (age 9-12)

- The King County Sexual Assault Resource Center in Washington State offers an excellent brochure entitled, *He Told Me Not To Tell: A parents' guide to talking to children about sexual assault'.* Call (425)226-5062 for a free copy

Index

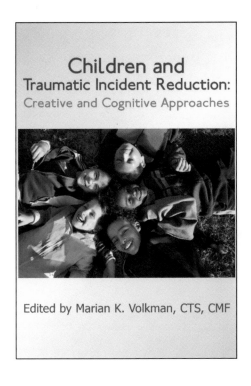

What if we could resolve childhood trauma early, rather than late?

We are understanding more and more about how early traumatic experiences affect long-term mental and physical health:

- Physical impacts are stored in muscles and posture
- Threats of harm are stored as tension
- Overwhelming emotion is held inside
- Negative emotional patterns become habit
- Coping and defense mechanism become inflexible

What if we could resolve childhood trauma before years go by and these effects solidify in body and mind?

In a perfect world, we'd like to be able to shield children from hurt and harm. In the real world, children, even relatively fortunate ones, may experience accidents, injury, illness, and loss of loved ones. Children unfortunate enough to live in unsafe environments live through abuse, neglect, and threats to their well-being and even their life.

Children And Traumatic Incident Reduction
ISBN 978-1-932690-30-9   List $19.95

More information at www.TIRbook.com

Sam Feels Better Now!
An Interactive Story

Sam saw something awful and scary! Ms. Carol, a special therapist will show Sam how to feel better. Children can help Sam feel better too by using drawings, play, and storytelling activities. They will be able to identify and manage their own feelings and difficulties in their lives following a traumatic event.

"This beautiful little picture book is the ideal guide for a series of therapy sessions that will focus the child's attention on positives and help to deal with the traumatic memories."

—Bob Rich, PhD.

"*Sam Feels Better Now* provides the child and therapist a safe metaphor for exploring trauma issues. The story teaches children that coming to therapy can be a good thing."

—JoAnna White, Ed.D., Chair, Department of Counseling and Psychological Services, Georgia State University

ISBN 978-1-932690-60-6   List $24.95

More information at www.JillOsborne.com

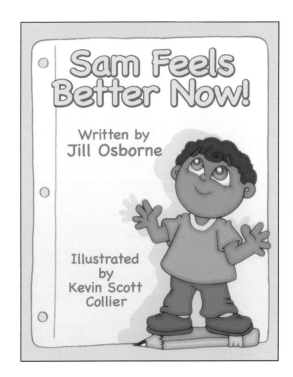

CPSIA information can be obtained
at www.ICGtesting.com
Printed in the USA
255247LV00005B